The Mi

By: Lanie Stevens

Legal Disclaimer:

The Miracle Mindset

Chapter 1 – Introduction

The subconscious mind is like a bank – a universal bank; it magnifies whatever you deposit or impress upon it." - Joseph Murphy

Do you believe in miracles? As a child you were probably more susceptible to believing in miracles but there are miracles all around you if you take a moment to appreciate them. In fact, you are a walking, talking, breathing, thinking miracle! The wonderment of life and the creation of a human from a sperm and an egg is a miracle. The fact that your body and mind can withstand years of neglect and abuse and survive an average of 86 years, if you are a female, is a miracle.

The fact that in your lifetime you will:

- Take 20,000 breaths a day or approximately 627,800,000 in a lifetime is a miracle;

- Have an average of 108,000 heartbeats a day or 39,420,000 a year is a miracle;

- The fact that you have an average of 50,000 thoughts a day – 80% being negative – 95% being repetitive is a miracle.

- Have approximately 18,250,000 thoughts a year and **17,337,500** of them being **the same thoughts you had the day before**!

You may wonder how you can possibly program yourself to manifest, using the Law of Attraction, when you are absentmindedly processing so many repetitive negative thoughts? And, obviously since they are the same negative thoughts as the day before they are mainly focused on the past with perhaps a few thoughts that are fretting over future negative events.

It is a *miracle* that you have manifested things in your life that are positive if you really think about it. As a child you expected miracles and you had a belief that you would be cared for, nurtured, protected and guided. You were innocent and had the luxury of trusting that life would turn out positively and you didn't even know the word "manifest". You felt indestructible because you hadn't lived long enough to experience disappointments, fear, rejection and loneliness. You could be fearless because you hadn't experienced failure.

As an adult you have years and years of disappointments, failures, resentments, lack, abandonment, worry, fear, health issues, loss, sadness, anger, jealousy and rejection. It's harder to let the things go that are holding you back and you simply file them away in your memory bank. Your memory bank is overflowing with life's experiences that you spend countless hours focusing on unintentionally. Most of them associated with negative emotions.

What if I told you that there is a method to once again attract the miracles you desire in your life with very little effort? They don't have to be huge miracles – *but they certainly have the potential to be.* Or, they may simply be the miracle of having money left over at the end of the month, finding a relationship that is fulfilling, learning a new style of connecting with your mate using mental telepathy, getting answers to your problems, being able to let go of the past to focus on the present or having extraordinary health. All are miracles in their own way – because they change your life!

"The Miracle Mindset" resets negative programming."

If you are one of the many, many people who have tried to use the Law of Attraction techniques without success, or with limited success, The Miracle Mindset may be the book for you. It will teach you simple and effective methods to shift your mindset, and let go of negative and repetitive thoughts, so you can more easily attract what you desire in life. You see, it isn't your fault that you keep attracting the things you don't want. It's the mindset and belief you've created *unintentionally* during your entire lifetime – without even realizing it!

This mindset is ingrained into your psyche because it began at birth, and continues till this day, and it affects everything in your life. You can't force the mindset to change – try as you may to do it – but you can cause it to positively shift by using this effective program.

Are you ready to shift your mindset? In this book you will learn how to:

- Stop sabotaging yourself and begin to attract more of what you desire;

- Clear out your subconscious baggage from as far back as childhood;

- Replace a defeated attitude with one of confidence;

- Attract and resonate with a compatible partner;

- Heal your body, mind and soul and create a healthy and energetic YOU;

- Live an inner and outer world of love, gratitude and peace;

- Have more self-esteem and self-worth than ever before;

- Resonate with the energy of wealth and financial security;

- Create a loving union with your mate through the power of your *entanglement*;

- Have a better sex life and marriage by strengthening your energetic connection;

- Initiate guidance and get answers from your subconscious or superconscious mind;

- Energetically connect with others using a specific technique;

- Live the life you desire to live!

You can simply *wish* for these things, and be disappointed when they don't show up, or you can begin to attract them into your life. If manifesting what you wanted in life were easy then everyone would live in a mansion, have maids, take fancy vacations and retire by age 40. But the fact is that we manifest every moment of every day by default and it is impossible to stop manifesting.

The good news is that, rather than spend a lifetime frustrated with your inability to manifest what you desire, you can begin today to program yourself for success! This book gives you all the information you need to shift your mindset to the miracle mindset if you follow the simple, easy-to-learn exercises. However, if you want a shortcut to successfully changing your life, and manifesting ability, without having to do *anything* but listen to powerful guided meditations as you go to bed at night you may want to check out the program I created available exclusively on my website. http://laniestevensauthor.com

Chapter 2 – Change Your Mindset

"It's not in the stars to hold our destiny –
but in ourselves."

I could just churn out relationship books on silly text message subjects, and probably make a fortune, but that isn't going to change your life in any way. I want more for you than just hoping for some small and insignificant event that will leave you ultimately feeling unsatisfied. I want to help you change what is blocking you from success in ALL areas of your life. Trust me, most people don't have a clue what that blockage is or how to overcome it!

This book is more than just another book on The Law of Attraction philosophy. It is designed to help you in every area of your life through specific methods where *you cannot fail*. It's more than just the *power of positive thinking*, having gratitude or living your life as if you already have what it is you desire. Although it is also doing some of those things, too.

If you are currently disenchanted with the mumbo-jumbo you've read about LOA, if you are looking for a program that teaches you how to succeed easily and effortlessly, if you desire to change your current financial status, your relationship, attract love, improve your health or *anything else you have complete control over* – this book can help you. And, it will help you in a short amount of time.

I'll bet you are one of many people who have jumped onto the LOA bandwagon only to abandon the idea the first time you failed at attracting something you desired. And, you're certainly not alone because more people fail than succeed because it's their mindset. *"It's not for me!"* is most likely what you declared when you tried to manifest something and were disappointed that you didn't get exactly what you desired. That only reinforced the failure of ALL the things you failed at in the past. Believe it or not, a half-hearted attempt at something is worse than not doing it at all! Your mind associates it with being a loser, not being able to succeed, and all of the other negative thoughts you have about yourself.

The Law of Attraction is a law that works perfectly 100% of the time just like the Law of Gravity. It's always working. It works by attracting to us what we are in alignment to receive. If you think of the universe as a giant ball of vibration and energy (which it is) you would see LOVE as the highest of all vibrations. You can't be in alignment with attracting love if you are in alignment with fear and a lack of love. When you are out of alignment with the thing you are seeking it is virtually impossible to attract *it* – whatever *it* may be.

"You attract what you are in alignment with energetically!"

Most people believe that it's the power of their conscious mind that controls their destiny. If it's simply *mind over matter* what happened in the cases where the last thing you wanted happened to show up? After all, you have probably thought positive thoughts, boosted that with a little prayer, perhaps negotiated with God (or some Higher Power) and did everything humanly possible to ensure that your wish would be granted. Your conscious mind is a pretty good negotiator.

When things don't turn out the way you want them to you may even make excuses like "I guess it wasn't meant to be" or "It probably turned out for the best". Thinking that at least if you could make yourself feel better about the failure you could better deal with it emotionally. Or so you believed.

You may listen to others' opinions or stories about how they've been faced with similar or even worse situations. Their lover left them, they lost their job, they have a debilitating health condition and they don't have a dime in the bank – but they have gratitude that things aren't even *worse* so they're going to try and stay positive. You may even be one of *those* people who occasionally look on the bright side of things regardless how dismal things may appear at the present moment. Or, you may be one of the people (some you may know) whose words don't match their inner belief. That's the true problem with manifesting the things you desire.

Yes, bad things happen to people who don't deserve it. But good things happen to people who know how to attain them. Whether they deserve them or not. However, before you can be open to receiving great things you must clear out the old, useless baggage you've been carrying around all your life.

There are many, many reasons you have probably given yourself as the reason(s) for leading a life that isn't quite living up to your expectations. YOU have the ability to change it. If you read Law of Attraction books it is *always* your fault that you haven't manifested your perfect life. And, there are many reasons suggested for your lack of success and they include:

- Not resonating on an energetic level;

- A predominance of thoughts you may be unaware of;

- Your *true* belief you have on the subject;

- The fact that you cannot trick your subconscious mind into believing through the direction of your conscious brain;

- That your visualizations lack something;

- Or any other reason that it is totally, **100% YOU**!

All of those things are true but you can't overcome and change them simply by recognizing them. There are programs running your life behind the scenes that sabotage you every moment of every day. You can't access them by *consciously* commanding them to change, you can't change them by *denying* their presence, you can't change them through *sheer will* – **but you can change them**!

You have been programmed at a *deep subconscious level* to attract what you now have in your life. It isn't a devious plan, scheme or the universe playing tricks on you. You aren't being intentionally singled out, deprived and made to live with less than you desire as some sort of strange punishment.

You don't fall in and out love with virtually the same person over and over again as a bad joke that the universe is playing on you. The person with the same personality traits, disposition, tendency to cheat or leave you when the going gets tough. The reason for the attraction isn't the bald head, or the controlling and narcissistic personality. It's that you are programmed to be attracted to a certain type of person through your experiences and the associations that the experiences have caused. Without you realizing it!

"Change your mindset – change your life!"

The truth of the matter is that you have been programmed since birth (and maybe in-utero) to believe certain things about yourself, life in general and your potential. It is the true problem with your manifestations, your choices in life and the issues with attracting positive experiences. Your inner mind, that subconscious mind that forgets nothing, has determined your value and your worth and it matches it with situations and people who are an energetic match.

It has a belief system about you based on input from others and your own personal beliefs about yourself. Personal beliefs that began at an early age and were influenced by your parents, your siblings, schoolmates, authority figures and everyone else. Beliefs that continued later in life and reinforced by your relationships, loves, spouse, friends and experiences. That's the magic of the unconscious mind to believe what is imprinted on it without questioning whether the input is valid.

That's also the issue when it is imprinted with false or negative thought beliefs. Your unconscious mind, that is responsible for approximately 90-95% of your choices, has been programmed to make decisions and attract things that negatively affect you.

Negative programming can cause:

- self-esteem issues;

- low expectations;

- unrealistic view regarding your worth and value;

- feelings of being unattractive;

- questioning your intelligence and choices;

- viewing yourself as inferior;

- health issues that are chronic or acute;

- insecurity in relationships;

- giving more than you receive;

- being taken advantage of in friendships & relationships;

- giving up your power to others;

- finding yourself in similar situations repeatedly;

- problems in relationships;

- many failed relationships;

- being promiscuous or frigid;

- never feeling fulfilled or truly happy;

- having a sense of dread or doom;

- suffering panic attacks or unexplained illnesses;

- having money issues;

- chronic depression;

- wanting to give up;

- afraid to ask for what you want;

- being accustomed to rejection;

- believing that you are a victim;

- accepting less than you deserve and desire.

Do you see yourself in any of the descriptions listed? All of these ideas about yourself were created through the power of your subconscious with the input you have received during your entire lifetime. If you have been made to feel *less than* during your lifetime you will resonate with things and people that treat you as *less than* you are. You can dress up, feel okay about yourself and present an outer appearance of confidence that will fool everyone you meet – but not the inner YOU. You can consciously tell yourself 10 times a day how beautiful, successful and lucky you are, and it will have *some effect*, but it will not fool the inner YOU and that is what needs to change before you can attract what you desire.

So how do you change this belief system that has been operating for 20, 30, 40 or 70 years? Believe it or not, it is pretty simple to do once you know how. Because the subconscious mind believes what you tell it as FACT all you have to do is reprogram it with the thoughts and *facts of your choosing*. You also must do it when your subconscious mind is receptive to the new ideas and that isn't done with your conscious mind. It is done through meditation and/or self-hypnosis because that's when you can get inside the subconscious mind to imprint new suggestions. The conscious mind isn't what's responsible for making changes or manifesting things into your life.

That's the reason you can't force yourself to change by making commands to your brain in your conscious state of mind! Your conscious mind absolutely hates change and, unless you trick it through hypnosis or meditation, your conscious mind will do anything possible to keep things status quo. So the *power of positive thinking* has to be at a deeper level than just your conscious mind attempting to direct your life through sheer force. We already know doesn't work.

Ask yourself these questions:

- How much time do you think you have left on this earth?

- How do you want to spend it?

- Is it worth trying a new program that will help you create a better life for the *rest of your life*?

- What do you have to lose?

You're going to live each day either choosing to make it differently or accepting it the way it is. And, you are manifesting every moment of every day whether you accept it as fact or not. Why not take control of your destiny and attract love, wealth, health and happiness learning exercises that can change your life.

Chapter 3 – Taking Control of Your Life

"You can't change what's going on around you until you change what's going on inside you."

Most women just want to get down to the important things in life – like meeting your soulmate and falling in love. However, the same energy to create a relationship exists in the creation of all things. Things like good health, wealth and happiness. Why not have them all instead of restricting it to just finding a mate? Remove the blockages that keep you from having a satisfying and fulfilling life in *all* areas.

I smile when I see books and receive questions about getting a text message from someone because I recognize it as two things:

    1. You don't have a belief that you deserve something more; and

2. You don't have faith and you need confirmation that LOA works without asking the universe for *too* much.

A text message isn't what you want! You want a real, honest, committed relationship and you believe a text is the first step because it's at least having contact with the person. Wrong! Accepting crumbs when you can have the whole cake isn't going to help your self-esteem or change your life. It will just reinforce the belief that you are not enough and you don't deserve anything more than crumbs. A message that you may have received inadvertently throughout your lifetime.

Unless you were lucky enough to be born into a home with devoted and loving parents who nurtured you, and were perfect and ideal specimens, you have a lot of negative programming to undo. Not placed there intentionally or maliciously but just due to life itself. Things happen and we internalize these things without consciously knowing it or being able to stop it from happening. You can't undo what you don't know you have. You have to recognize it to begin to change it!

How does negative programming affect you? It keeps you living in a lower vibrating energy for one thing. That low vibration seeks its' own level and keeps things status quo. The negative mindset is part of your subconscious mind, the mind that forgets nothing and remembers and categorizes everything. It is a very efficient computer that has perfect recall. So how do we get what we want in life without struggling and feeling like each and every day is an uphill battle? Once you recognize without a doubt that your conscious brain isn't what manifests your desires it's easier to direct the part of your brain that does – the subconscious mind.

The subconscious mind operates below your normal level of consciousness and it is busily working behind the scenes as it controls your breathing, your heartbeat, your hormones, your nervous system, your beliefs, what you attract and basically everything! It also absorbs or rejects information based on your perception of the world around you. If the information you received during your childhood (and adulthood) was incorrect, or negative, your subconscious has a view of the world that may be skewed. It's hard to attract anything but the same old stuff if you're still wired with negative and faulty wiring. After all, your subconscious mind remembers literally everything you've experienced in life! Thoughts, feelings and emotions!

By the time you were a child of 6-7 years old your subconscious mind received input that still impacts you NOW. Parents who were neglectful, chaotic, unloving or who lacked empathy may have told you or implied that you were stupid, unimportant, unlovable, lazy or a burden – and these messages may still impact you at a level beneath your level of awareness. Even if you had perfect parents (highly unlikely) you most likely had other encounters at school, with siblings or friends who placed negative feedback in your unconscious memory bank. Your memory bank, that subconscious mind, is full of programs that decide your fate and luck and it remembers everything (good and bad) that has happened to you from birth up to the present time. Not only that it has the stored emotions associated with the memories.

"Negative programming happens ALL during your life!"

It doesn't even have to be just from childhood that you've been programmed because it happens all during your lifetime. I'm sure you can remember incidents that happened years ago that still bring hurt, sadness, embarrassment, feelings of inferiority or insecurity and a pain so deep inside that the feelings resurface as if it just happened yesterday. I'm not going to ask you to remember those times, but I guarantee you there are memories that still ignite feelings you'd rather not remember or experience. To remember them would make you feel as if you were experiencing them at the present moment and it would most likely create a powerful response.

The negative programs are always ready to be accessed and they are what make you prone to have accidents, failed relationships, bad luck, illnesses, lack of love and money and other negative experiences. The same can be said of the good experiences in life because a positive mindset will bring you good luck, fortune, happiness and success. Most of the time you operate on auto-pilot, and very little attention is paid to training your mind for success, so your luck is influenced by negative external stimulation rather than internal direction.

An example of negative programming happened when I was visiting a friend of mine one day many years ago. Her 6-year-old daughter loved to sing and she was happily singing while I was sitting and chatting with my girlfriend. Suddenly, and without warning, my friend told her to "hush her singing because she had a horrible voice". I was literally dumbfounded and later addressed it with my friend. She defended herself by saying "I am just tired of hearing her sing all the time" but she recognized that she had been extremely harsh.

Although she hugged her daughter, and apologized profusely, the damage had been done and that statement caused her daughter to never sing again. Her daughter, now 24-years-old, recently visited and I mentioned her beautiful voice and how I loved to listen to her sing when she was a child. She emphatically stated that she never liked to sing because her voice was "horrible", and I could tell she still seemed sensitive about the subject. That memory has been held in her subconscious mind for 18 years, and it has impacted her view of herself, but she has no conscious memory of the incident.

You may find you have difficulty in certain areas of your life and you just can't find your groove enough to change it. You may be unsure of what it is, but there is something playing behind the scenes that you can't quite grasp, and it doesn't allow you to achieve the success you desire. It can be in relationships, business or any other area that you received, or continue to receive, these messages that lead you astray and stop your success. The programming never stops! You will take information and impressions you receive from your outer world and internalize them all during your life. What does your subconscious do with these messages?

It associates them! For instance, let's say you were in a relationship that you thought was really going somewhere and suddenly out of the blue he dropped you, you broke up, or he abandoned you and that rejection rocked your world to its' core. Your conscious brain may try to rationalize or go over and over the *facts* as it seeks to uncover an answer. But your subconscious mind will associate this rejection with other similar ones in the past. You know, the time your friend made plans with you and then changed them at the last minute when they got a better offer? Your parents getting a divorce and the feelings of abandonment. A childhood memory of having very few friends you could count on. Or perhaps a parent who neglected to be there for you when you really, really needed them. Maybe another old relationship that may not have outright rejected you but just slowly faded away until you were left wondering what the hell happened.

It doesn't just make you feel rejected. It also associates the incidents with feelings about yourself that may include untrue beliefs such as: you are unlovable, disposable, unattractive, undesirable, unloved, unappreciated, or just have a sense of *not being enough*. It doesn't matter that these beliefs are untrue even if you are told that over and over again by well-meaning friends or family that you are wonderful and an amazing person. That association stays in your subconscious until you change the association and reprogram your mindset.

You can't push the association away into the recesses of your mind because the memories are already there in the recesses of your mind, and they will remain there, until you replace or diffuse them. In fact, your subconscious mind is the mind of remembrance. While your conscious mind remembers and recalls some things it is your subconscious mind that has *total* recall. Every detail of every moment of your life. With no exception. And, all of those memories have feelings associated with them because that's how your subconscious mind operates – feelings.

I don't usually share this with others, but I was sexually molested from the time I was about 4 until the age of approximately 9. I rejected the memories of that molestation and totally shut down that part of my life consciously. In doing so I really couldn't remember anything about those 5 years of my childhood whether good or bad. However, my subconscious mind remembered every detail. How did I figure it out?

I have always been fascinated with the power of the mind so I went to someone years ago who, through hypnosis, took me back to that time in my life. Strangely enough I went to a hypnotherapist because I was unable to listen to football games without experiencing a deep, deep sadness. A sadness that was so all encompassing it would ruin my weekends and I would end up in bed crying or sleeping all day. I had no idea why football games would have such an overwhelming and negative impact on me but I decided to try hypnosis to find out. It worked!

I discovered that as a child I was molested in a closet that had a common wall with a room that had a TV playing football games. While having no conscious memory of that time my subconscious mind remembered every detail and I was able to clear out the association and move forward in my life and rid myself of the debilitating sadness I had experienced. I even go to football games and/or watch them now with no lingering feelings of despair. Not only that but I was able to get back the years of repressed memories of my childhood and could even remember the name of students in my classroom as well as the teacher's name.

Your subconscious mind forgets *nothing* and catalogs *everything*.

So how can you get rid of old negative thoughts and wounds so you can begin to attract what you desire? Releasing the past and changing your mindset from one of failure and misery to one of happiness and joy. You can go to a hypnotherapist who is qualified to take you back to your childhood and spend thousands of dollars and years of your life, or you can do it the easy way. The way I will teach you where you can easily help yourself without years of therapy or time. I want you to take control of your life so you won't waste countless years experiencing pain, suffering, lack or loss. It is my desire for you to live your best life possible by changing your mindset to win in every area of your life. Where miracles are an everyday occurrence and they are to be expected – not something that happens only to other people – but something that happens to YOU!

Chapter 4 – Who is Responsible?

"You may believe that you are responsible for what you do, but not for what you think. The truth is that you are responsible for what you think, because it is only at this level that you can exercise choice. What you do comes from what you think." -- Marianne Williamson

You are responsible for everything in your life. Haven't you heard that statement many, many times before in every Law of Attraction book you've ever read? You need to take responsibility for the love affair that's gone badly, the job with the boss you despise, the unappreciative children you've raised, the dog who craps behind the chair instead of outside, the never-ending housework, the weight you've gained due to the rise of cortisol in your over-worked body, the stress of living paycheck to paycheck, the husband who is a lazy douche, and the unpaid bills that are jamming up your mailbox -- YEP, it's all you! You've manifested it through the power of your thoughts only you can't remember thinking or wishing these things upon yourself. Who would do that?

It has nothing to do with the fact that life is life and at best it's more difficult than not. Most of us are just average, ordinary people who struggle with the day to day stresses we encounter. We don't have the time, money or guidance necessary to change things because we are just too busy just surviving. Our conscious brain runs our daily lives because it is the brain of survival. It can't seem to see the forest from the trees but without it you may forget to pay your bills, take the meatloaf out of the oven or pick the kids up at school. I mean you do need that conscious brain to take care of everyday tasks. But you don't need that conscious brain to have control of your life!

Can you help it if that conscious brain is mentally spewing *gibberish* nonsense to you 24/7 and, even if you tried, you just can't seem to turn it off? It's like the damn thing has a mind all its' own and all it wants to think about is the past and all the hardships, resentments, pain and injustices it has endured and – even worse, it makes you relive all those events. Over and over and over and over again.

It even takes you back to childhood as it associates things in the present with things in the past. Yes, your husband is exactly like your alcoholic father who never showed affection. His temper explodes just like dear ole' Dad's where you had to walk on eggshells for fear of making him mad. You are turning into your mother just like you feared and those memories of her come back when you speak to your own children. When you're not invited to a function it brings back memories of feeling alone and rejected by your peers. You're afraid to show your displeasure with your mate for fear that he will abandon you. The slightest and smallest present-day memory will trigger those memories of years ago. Whether good or bad – well, mostly bad.

It doesn't focus so much on the present or the positive and good times you've experienced. If it isn't focusing on the past it wants you to fear the future. Your thoughts may be of all the things you have to fear that may kill you, harm your children, make your husband run off, put bacteria in your food, subject you to dangerous situations in some way and ultimately endanger or snuff out your life. When awake your brain is always on active mode and it is usually focusing on the things you don't want to think about. Like things that bring you harm emotionally and physically or associations that you would rather bury deep and never remember again.

Your conscious brain wants you to survive the conundrum called life in the only way it knows how --

and that way is to allow fear and negativity to take over as a way to protect you. It doesn't do it to harm you, make your life miserable or take the fun out of life. It does it because it's programmed to live at any cost. Who programmed your brain? You did. All throughout your life, in every experience (real or imagined), every memory, every visualization and every belief – you have created your reality. Your conscious brain is a born fighter, fighting for life and survival, but your subconscious mind remembers every detail of your life and it is programmed to attract things to you that have impacted you the most *emotionally.*

Negative events and memories tend to have a longer lasting effect on us because there is more emotion involved! Sure, you remember things of great importance like your wedding day, the birth of a child, the day you were promoted or the first time you laid eyes on your mate. But those aren't the memories you focus on, are they? Instead you have more emotion around disappointments, failures, slights, resentment, upsets or fears – and, those are the memories you keep going over and over in your mind. Not the positive ones – the negative ones!

There is a part of your brain that will keep you breathing even when doctors have pronounced you brain dead unless that part of your brain was severely injured. It is simply the way your conscious brain is wired from birth – to survive. Try as you may to change it you are simply at its' mercy most of the time. You are a prisoner of unwanted thoughts and, even if you tried, you cannot turn the thoughts off. Imagine having approximately 50,000 thoughts a day with the majority of them recalling negative incidents in your life and up to 90% of those thoughts being repetitive. So, day after day after day you obsess over things that unsurface negative emotions. It is living in a world of pollution!

Where the hell did that negative chatterbox, slightly berserk brain come from anyway? Who wants to listen to it and how can you stop it? So, this is the thing that creates your reality according to the Law of Attraction, huh? This brain that attracts all the bad situations, people and results into your life that you have no conscious control over. It's like trying to stop a grenade from detonating by holding one finger over it and thinking it into disintegrating. Or, to control a runaway train by standing in front of it. Not being able to control your thoughts is bad enough but now you are actually being blamed by Law of Attraction gurus saying that it is all your *fault*. That's definitely insult to injury.

I don't know about you but trying to train your conscious brain into having an ounce of gratitude or peace when someone cuts you off in traffic *and* shoots you the finger, or when you need to rush back to work after lunch and the slowpokes in the food line are chatting about the weather, or when a salesperson is rude and clearly doesn't want to wait on you, or when your mate picks a fight for no reason, or your children are trashing your freshly cleaned home – is damn near impossible. Peace and happiness? You've gotta be kidding me!

If it were that easy to control your life through the *power of positive thinking* why aren't you a multi-millionaire living a grand life on an island somewhere with butlers, maids and a gourmet cook? After all, sometimes you do think positive thoughts so that should count for something! You think perhaps your negative thoughts are to blame for your life of lack. You're cognizant that your conscious brain does focus on a lot of negative thoughts it conjures up. Is that why you continue to attract things you don't desire? Because you are in alignment with negativity rather than positivity?

Trying to police the negative thoughts and separate them into categories of negative and positive is a feat for *Rainman,* the hit movie that featured Dustin Hoffman as an idiot savant. He was brilliant with numbers but had no common sense whatsoever. His brain was highly functioning but on only one aspect – numbers. You would need to be a savant to count and categorize your thoughts to figure out whether you had more positive, more negative or more neutral thoughts and determine how they have affected your life.

"Only 5% of conscious thoughts impact what you manifest!"

If you have that much time on your hands a *"mani/pedi"* would probably be more satisfying emotionally than wasting time focusing even more intensely on your conscious brain. The good news is that it is estimated that your conscious brain is responsible for only about 5% or less in manifesting. Those random, irritating and annoying thoughts, that you can't get rid of no matter how hard you try, don't stick around long enough in your consciousness to generate the emotion necessary for actual manifestation. I mean when you have up to how 18 million thoughts a year how could you manifest into reality that many things? It is illogical and impossible.

The thoughts that do manifest are the ones you obsess over and place a lot of emotion into!

So how do we change our circumstances if it isn't through our conscious brain? Aren't there thousands of best-selling books out there about the *power of positive thinking*? If they didn't work why would they be selling like hotcakes? I look at it this way – if you could actually change your reality by *simply* changing your thoughts why are there so many people still stuck in mundane lives? It isn't that people don't attempt to live their lives in a manner that positively affects others so at least their karma should be kicking in and make up for the lack of positive thinking.

The majority of people are relatively generous whether it is with money, love, time or affection so those are all positive actions and feelings. Unless you rob houses, rape and pillage (doubtful) or wish evil crap on others I'm sure you should be reaping some rewards somewhere. So why hasn't your life of 30, 40, 50 or 80 years changed very much? Why have you been stuck on the merry-go-round of the *"do unto others as they do unto you"* belief and philosophy and yet you continue to struggle?

You most likely haven't won the lottery, although I'm sure you've tried, and you're probably still working or retired and on a budget. You may be in a relationship but aren't quite happy with the current status quo or perhaps you're seeking *the one* and have thought you've found him many, many times only to find out he's a loser or has a fear of commitment. You may experience exhaustion or a list of health issues that you don't have time to address. So, when does the karmic *blessing bank* open up and spill out upon you all of the many things you should have saved up due to your kindness, generosity, karma, positivity and the fact that you haven't killed someone – lately? When does the *power of positive thinking* kick in?

Your blessings are there and waiting for you and they always has been. You just haven't known how to get your blessings out of the bank they've been saved in. View it as that old-fashioned piggy bank that had the slit in the top for you to put money into. You have been saving for all these years, but you haven't been able to take your money (good fortunes) out of it. You may have tried shaking the bank hoping something would accidentally fall out of it. But you never knew there was a secret opening at the bottom because you never turned it over and inspected it.

Just like your life. You live your life the same old way – day in and day out – hoping that one day something good is going to fall out of it. Some rich, handsome prince is going to ride up in his white limo. Your lottery numbers will be chosen and you'll be the next billionaire. You'll have as much health and energy as you did when you were a young child. After all, you've put a lot of years into life, and have tried to be the best person possible, so why don't you have all the riches and blessings that life has to offer?

The fact is that your good fortune is waiting for you as soon as you get your beliefs about yourself in alignment to receive it. A relationship, financial gain, health for yourself and others and even a connection that can answer your questions and guide you along your path – **all within your reach**. They are there and they always have been. You just didn't have access to your treasures. Gratitude, peace, positive thinking? Yes, you will experience those things when you begin to change your life. Hopefully that journey for you will begin today.

Chapter 5 – Subconscious Mind Facts

There have been many attempts to control and reset the brain and most of have failed miserably. For instance, how many people do you know who have gone through years and years of talk therapy re-hashing, *and possibility reinforcing*, the trauma they are trying to rid themselves of to no avail. Training the brain through conscious programming and commands has been tried, too. But trying to change things that are programmed into the subconscious cannot be undone by *forcing* it through control. If that could be accomplished then lives would be much simpler because it would simply be a *mind over matter* issue.

In the not so distant past teachers would make students write negative statements over and over again as punishment for some violation. This would only imprint the subject even more into the subconscious mind and the negative programming would be reinforced. At least now it is recognized that positive affirmations leave a positive imprint on the subconscious although it's not a very strong impression in and of itself. But it is an improvement!

Many years ago electric shock therapy was used to help people who were suicidal, bipolar or suffered severe depression and it was thought to short circuit or restart and reset the brain. Although still used it isn't as severe and unregulated as it once was and now it's been proven to help serotonin levels and raise other chemicals in your body to help fight depression. Basically, it is your body and mind resetting the old programming. I know people who have had this treatment done to them.

A friend of mine was almost electrocuted when she was about 12 years old when she touched an ungrounded light bulb while standing in water. Yeah, I know, not very smart but she was only 12. She had so much electricity running through her body she couldn't let go of the bulb and she still remembers that her entire life was flashing like pictures through her mind. It was as if her subconscious mind, which relates to pictures and feelings, was playing out her life as if she were watching a movie and in a matter of a few seconds time. Your memories are recorded, and they are there for your entire lifetime – whether you are 12 years old or 100 years old.

You may ask if it's possible to change and correct old negative patterns and programs and the answer is – absolutely, positively, without a doubt **YES**! When you begin to reprogram old thought patterns and replace them with new, powerful, positive beliefs your life will begin to shift from lack to bountiful. You can also do some things yourself to eliminate unwanted negativity that affects your subconscious mind and I highly recommend starting by consciously doing these simple things:

- Make your environment a positive and stress-free one. Watch less crime shows, news and horror movies to limit the negativity being absorbed into your subconscious mind. Remember, your subconscious believes what it sees and feels as real and it doesn't have the ability to filter it!

- Limit your time with negative people and surround yourself with people who are positive, have a good outlook on life and you enjoy being around. Stay away from "energy vampires" who drain your energy and dump all of their problems on you. Take inventory now of those "friends".

- Use the 3 second rule! When you have an unpleasant, unrelenting negative thought allow yourself only 3 seconds to acknowledge it before shifting your focus intentionally and replacing it with a positive experience, thought or emotion.

- Your subconscious mind thrives on pictures and visualizations so reprogram it with 10-15 minutes of meditation a day. It works miracles! Immerse yourself in your visualizations and try to engage all of your senses as you allow joy, peace and happiness sensations to flood your body. The exercises in the book are an excellent way to begin!

- Read or listen to affirmations and allow yourself to have the corresponding feelings. If your affirmation is "I am in a relationship" and you feel alone, and like a loser, it isn't going to work. Repetition is key so say them to yourself over and over again. And, do it throughout the day.

- Meditate yourself to sleep at night while listening to music designed to relax and calm your mind. It's the perfect time to reset your brain for positivity.

All of these suggestions will help you to consciously, from this day forward, change your mindset. But what about the past decades that still affect you? Is there a way to rid yourself of the past without years of hypnotherapy and reliving all of the incidents that are still there clogging up your subconscious mind? Absolutely!

"Your subconscious mind has perfect recall!"

First, let's look at some facts about your subconscious that you may find interesting:

- Your subconscious mind is a world of *thought, feeling* and *power;*

- It controls approximately 90-95% of your reality;

- It has infinite wisdom, power and the ability to create and manifest what you desire;

- All achievement and all success come directly from that hidden power within;

- Creating harmony within creates an environment and energy resonance for manifestation;

- Your subconscious also has the ability to create distress, sickness, lack, discord and limitation when it is in disharmony;

- It is through the subconscious mind that you can connect to others, as well as to the Universal Mind, because we are all connected through what quantum physics refers to as *entanglement*;

- Every thought and feeling creates a *cause and effect* so controlling your thoughts and emotions changes your physical outcome and manifestation;

- To remove any subconscious discord you must change your mindset and your outer world will positively change;

- There is an infinite supply of energy and blessings by tapping into the Universal mind;

- The subconscious is the mind of creation and creativity so when you are directed by it -- follow it;

- The subconscious is automatically engaged while your conscious brain is functioning. Things like driving or playing an instrument while having a conversation shows how your brains work in conjunction;

- It remembers everything and it is awake 24/7;

- It is our memory bank for names, faces, facts, thoughts and even visualization;

- Ever wake up in the middle of the night from a sound sleep? Yes, it's your ever awake subconscious mind warning you of possible danger;

- It automatically takes care of bodily functions such as breathing, heartrate, metabolism, and the millions of functions necessary for life to continue;

- It relies on your conscious mind to guard it from mistaken impressions;

- False suggestions to the subconscious can cause them to materialize. They include: poverty, disease, fear, worry, doom, depression, etc.;

- When your subconscious perceives something as truth it will *immediately* begin to act upon the impression;

- The subconscious can be influenced by others to become fearful, have poor self-image, be greedy, be distressed, negative, feel unworthy, etc.;

- It perceives instantly using intuition rather than conscious reasoning;

- It is where your aspirations reside and thrive;

- You can reprogram negative programming by overcoming them with a *stronger and more productive suggestion.* Repeated frequently the subconscious will accept the new suggestion;

- It is the *seat of the soul* and the connection to the Divine.

As you can see the subconscious mind is essential to utilizing the Law of Attraction effectively. The subconscious mind is what you will positively influence using this program. Your subconscious mind will do exactly what you direct it to do without discernment once you learn how to command it. Utilizing some simple exercises, you will begin to take command your subconscious mind and your life will begin to change.

Chapter 6 – Your Self-Concept

"Your subconscious mind makes all of your words and actions fit a pattern consistent with your self-concept and your innermost beliefs about yourself." - Brian Tracy

You can fool others with your outer appearance and actions, but you cannot fool your subconscious mind. Are your innermost thoughts and beliefs about yourself reflected in the following statements or something just as negative and disempowering?

- Why is my life so difficult;

- Why do I attract the same type of mate;

- Why can't I get ahead financially;

- Why am I such a loser;

- Things will never get better;

- I'm physically and emotionally exhausted;

- What is causing my illnesses;

- Why is money always an issue;

- I can never seem to attract positive things;

- I am doomed to failure;

- It's not me – it's my mate that's the problem;

- I have no control over my life and relationships;

- What is wrong with ME?

If so, you are fighting against subconscious programs that are running your life without your knowledge. It's like trying to run from the past while being handcuffed to it! You cannot change your future without programming yourself for success through re-programming your subconscious mind. It is virtually impossible!

Remember, your subconscious mind is the mind of acceptance. It accepts whatever you tell it to believe as FACT. Without questions, without reservations, without any proof – your thoughts and beliefs are taken as 100% fact! But it goes deeper than that. It doesn't just accept the facts that your conscious brain tells it to believe. No, that would be too simple. If it did you could just overpower your subconscious with the *power of positive thinking* and be hugely successful by now through your conscious thoughts.

Your subconscious mind accepts what it believes to be *facts* based on your innermost belief system, visualizations and experiences. Watch a horror film and you will feel your heartrate go up and the fear inside you increase automatically. Why? Your subconscious brain believes what you are watching is real and it causes your body to react! It experiences it as something happening to you and not simply a movie that is non-threatening although you know, on a rational level, it isn't real.

When I watched the movie *Scream* I couldn't walk outside alone to my car for a month! My conscious mind knew it wasn't real, and I wasn't in danger, but my subconscious mind still believed I was in dire danger. The same is true when I watch alien stuff. I know consciously I'm not going to be taken on a spacecraft and implanted with a weird device but my subconscious, based entirely on my fear and imagination, is convinced that I'm in danger. And, it is based entirely on my vivid internal visualizations.

"Your subconscious mind believes ANYTHING you impress upon it without questioning!"

So consciously trying to program yourself in a waking state isn't very effective ultimately. Your waking state isn't where the miracles happen because your conscious brain CANNOT program your unconscious brain without getting it into a relaxed, altered state.

If you could *consciously* force yourself to believe through sheer willpower, then the millions and millions of people who use the Law of Attraction religiously would be successful in every area of their lives. My readers' biggest complaint and questions about using the Law of Attraction is that they *want* to believe but they just can't *force* themselves. The mind over matter isn't working and deep down inside there is a belief that stops the manifesting in its' tracks. It isn't their fault! It's the fault of the programming and input they have received over their entire lifetimes.

Because I counsel women, mostly about relationships, I find that women will attract the same man with a different face and body over and over again. Even though the previous relationships were never what they desired and weren't satisfying. They try to make new relationships work but it's impossible. Then they wonder what they have done wrong and want advice on how they can fix the problem with *them*.

It isn't that they consciously pick the same type person that they were never really that attracted to, or truly in alignment with, in the first place. It's that their programming has made them settle for someone with certain characteristics that fall into what is comfortable for them. Comfortable to them because it fits into the programming of their unconscious mind. Men who may ignore them, feel superior, be unavailable emotionally, cheat on them, disregard their feelings, make them feel insignificant, mistreat them, use them or end up leaving them.

The conscious mind would reject these men immediately because it would recognize the warning signs, having experienced them before, consider the outcome and not let the relationship develop. The unconscious mind says:

- This is what I accept will happen;

- Abandonment will happen sooner or later;

- All men have treated me this way;

- It must be something I deserve;

- I am unworthy of something better;

- I can change them and the outcome if I try harder;

- They must be a more valuable person than I am;

- For some reason I am attracted to *bad boys*;

- Men cheat and I should expect and accept it.

Trying to figure out where that negative programming came from is like looking for the proverbial *needle in a haystack*. And, it doesn't really matter. It could have been an alcoholic and absent father, a mother who cared very little, feeling insignificant, a lack of childhood friends, little emotional support or abandonment issues (real or imagined). Or, none or ALL of these reasons. All that matters is that the programming is there, it has been there and will continue to be there, until YOU do something to change it!

Your brain is like a child and it will obey your commands if you present them in the correct manner. Trying to give a disobedient and willful child a command while they are in the middle of a temper tantrum doesn't work so well. Giving commands to your conscious and/or subconscious brain while fully awake and alert doesn't work very well, either. So, in order to begin reprogramming you should be in an "alpha" state. This is the state where you are relaxed, peaceful and calm and you may feel as if space and time are altered. The receptive state for meditation, visualizations and affirmations. This is the perfect time to re-program and trick your subconscious mind into *believing* a new reality. It doesn't matter if the reality is a visualization or verbal commands, that aren't true, because your subconscious mind will still believe every word you *say* or *see*.

Your "beta" state is your normal, active, alert, waking state where you are thinking and reacting. It is virtually impossible to re-program yourself in this state. When you are in the "theta" state there are exercises you can do to get answers to questions, see images or increase your psychic powers. This is the state you enter into right before you fall asleep at night and it is wonderful for meditation and hypnosis. By the way, there is no difference between guided meditations and hypnosis. They are both designed to implant suggestions and affirmations into your subconscious mind. Meditation without guidance will be calming but it is not designed to influence your subconscious mind.

Your "delta" state is when you are sound asleep and resting and your physical body is healing, resetting and restoring.

Years of negative thoughts and programming can be undone with some simple steps as you fall asleep at night. For this reason, I have created a program to help you become successful in all areas of your life and it is available only on my website. All the work has been done for you in this program and all you have to do is listen to the MP3 recordings as you fall asleep at night. Or, you can create a program of your own with the information you'll receive in the exercises in the following chapters.

Whether you are trying to manifest a mate, get a better paying job, attract wealth, become healthier and slimmer or even access your own psychic powers – you can do so easily when you reprogram or *deprogram* your subconscious mind and begin to create a miracle mindset.

Chapter 7 – Programming for Alpha State

> *"It is almost impossible to be consistent with your goal if your subconscious mind is constantly fed with negative perceptions of its' road."* – Edmond Mbiaka

From the earlier chapters you know that the alpha state is the perfect state of mind to be in when you want to impress the subconscious mind with new ideas, beliefs, affirmations and thoughts. It is achieved through shifting your mind from your outer world into the inner world through meditation and visualization.

This simple, easy exercise will begin to program your subconscious mind to go into an alpha state easily and effortlessly. It will also implant a suggestion to your subconscious mind that *every time* you begin this exercise it will shift into the state of reprogramming and preparation for suggestions of *change*.

Repetition is key so do the exercise each night before sleep. You will begin to look forward to it as the perfect end to your day. This particular exercise is getting your subconscious mind accustomed to going into the alpha state easily and with very little effort on your part. By simply stating the word "*sleep*" to yourself at the beginning of each exercise you will begin to shift your consciousness automatically. It's the shortcut and fastest way to reach the state of total relaxation and the place where you can let go of the past and re-program with affirmations.

EXERCISE FOR ENTERING ALPHA STATE

1. When you get into bed and are ready for sleep try this simple exercise. Close your eyes and breathe in to the count of 4, hold the breath to the count of 7, breathe out to the count of 8. Do this several times but don't make yourself dizzy. This will immediately begin to relax you.

2. Now visualize a golden staircase in your mind's eye. This staircase may be illuminating a golden light and it just has steps going **DOWN** right in front of you. Don't try to overthink this and wonder what's holding the staircase in place. Just

visualize the staircase as you are relaxing and visualizing.

3. See the stairs in front of you and notice that you seem to magically float down as you count the stairs. You aren't exercising any effort, you aren't stepping on the rungs, you are just floating down as you begin to count. With every step you take **DOWN** say the word "*sleep*" in your mind. Start with the number 15, visualize or mentally repeat the word *sleep* as you count down very slowly. 15, 14, 13, 12, 11,......

4. As you continue to descend keep focusing on the stairs. During a guided visualization I will have you picture the numbers in front of you and then the numbers fade away. They may be in a cloud or wisp or just a brightly lit number and then a fading number. You can try that visualization if you would like or mentally create one of your own that works for you.

5. Keep counting very slowly until you reach the number zero. If you are doing the counting slowly enough you will have enough time to completely and totally relax

and focus your attention. If it's not enough time or you feel anxious start at a higher number and count DOWN.

6. Once you reach the number zero do the following:

- Say the word *"sleep"* over and over again slowly for 30 seconds to a minute. As you say the word really feel how good it feels to relax completely. Feel the pleasant sensation and give the intention to remember the feeling and place it in your memory bank for future recall.

- Make a mental command for your mind to keep the command *"sleep"* in your memory bank permanently AND forever whenever you need to go into the alpha state;

- Repeat the statement a few times to implant it firmly into your subconscious.

7. After you have done this make the command IT IS DONE or simply LET THIS

COMMAND BE FULFILLED. You may then begin to count UP until you reach the number you started with and you will be ready for sleep.

Whatever you do please don't turn on the television, read or do anything else when you have finished with the programming because it negates the effect. Try to just relax and go to sleep. In my guided meditations there is music that plays (for a total of one hour) and messages that continue that alternate from the right to the left ear so both sides of the brain are entrained. However, if you are doing it on your own just either fall asleep or listen to gentle meditative music.

Since you are incapable of thinking of two things at the same time the fact that you are continuing to count after your mental *sleep* command you will give your subconscious mind time to absorb the message and begin to retrain your brain. Your subconscious mind is reprogrammed when you are consistent and repetitive with the programming. Do it every night for at least 3 nights then the program will change.

Chapter 8 – Programming to Relax

"Busy your mind with the concepts of harmony, health, peace and good will and wonders will happen in your life."

How many years you have listened to the same old program in your mind? Your inner mind knows the answer. I know that it is possible to change that programming very quickly using this program. To negate old programming you simply replace it with something else. The key is to do it over and over again until it overrides the old program. That's why it's best to do it at night as you are ready to fall asleep. You will train your conscious mind that when you get into bed it is time to retrain your brain.

I have a little Maltese who is 3 years old. Lolly and I have a routine that she learned very early on and that is when I turn the lights off in my living room she runs into the bedroom, twirls 3-4 times letting me know she's ready for bed, I lean over to pick her up as she turns her rear-end towards me and she then jumps onto the bed from my arms. She then gets into the same spot she always sleeps in and goes to sleep. This happens every single night!

"Rewire your brain for happiness through meditation and repetition!"

My point is that the same thing happens with your subconscious mind when you create a routine and expectation. It will begin to happen automatically. Because I meditate in bed my body and mind shift into a different space just by the act of getting into my bed. It can be during the day or at night. It is an intention that I set consciously as a trigger for my subconscious. To shift your current reality you must create a space of comfort and repetition. It can be a favorite chair, your bed or any other place of comfort and quiet. Just keep it the same each and every time if possible. The repetition will cause things to shift much faster than occasional meditations and visualizations or doing it at different times and places. A few minutes each and every day is more effective than a few hours of continuous meditation once a week!

Eventually it will happen so automatically you will be on auto-pilot when it comes to making huge changes in your life. You can shift your inner world, and make major shifts in your outer world, but you must do it consistently. The better you become at visualization and relaxation the faster your results will be – guaranteed.

For this exercise I just simply want you to relax your body one part at a time. Why do this? When your body is completely and totally relaxed it becomes ready for suggestions and/or affirmations. You can't be successful doing this to your conscious mind because it will resist it, analyze it and reject it. Only your subconscious mind will make the changes you desire in your life.

Begin by doing the same steps as before with the "*sleep*" exercise:

EXERCISE TO RELAX YOUR BODY

1. When you get into bed and are ready for sleep close your eyes and breathe in to the count of 4, hold the breath to the count of 7, breathe out to the count of 8. Do this several times but don't make yourself dizzy. This will immediately begin to relax you.

2. Tell yourself *sleep* a few times. Since you have been doing the exercise for a few days you should immediately shift into a relaxed and receptive state. If you find you haven't relaxed enough do the exercise (steps 1-5) from the previous chapter until you reach the bottom of the staircase but don't start back up the staircase, yet.

3. Once you are totally relaxed it's time to relax your body one body part at a time. Take your time because this exercise should last at least 10-15 minutes. Start at the top of your head as you start your relaxation and breathe gently allowing your body to fully relax. Top of head, scalp, forehead, eyes, jaw, neck, shoulders, arms, fingertips, spine, chest muscles, tummy, lower back, buttocks, thighs, knees, ankles and toes. Really focus on them and visualize them relaxing totally and completely. You may feel yourself getting very relaxed and sleepy – that's a great sign it's working.

4. Now make a mental command for your mind to keep the feeling of total relaxation in your memory bank permanently AND forever and

state this a few times to implant it firmly into your subconscious.

5. After you have done this make the command IT IS DONE or simply LET THIS COMMAND BE FULFILLED. You may then allow yourself to fall asleep if possible.

6. Do this exercise for 3 days before going on to the next exercise to ensure that you can totally and completely relax. It will get easier and easier to do as you continue to train your subconscious mind.

As before you will be ready for sleep so it's best if you don't turn on the television, read or do anything else that's distracting. Allow the feeling of relaxation to really permeate your cells because this is a very healing exercise and it is creating the feeling you need in order to begin the reprogramming exercises. There is no better way to heal your body, mind and soul than relaxation from head to toe. If you have the ability to visualize or imagine each body part letting go of tension, pressure, illness or stress this is the time to practice!

I also focus on my internal organs individually to get the most benefit from the exercise. You can visualize them one-by-one and *see* the healing light penetrating into the cells. When you intentionally send energy to your organs they respond instantly.

Chapter 9 – Releasing Negative Emotions

Forgiving does not erase the bitter past. A healed memory is not a deleted memory. Instead, forgiving what we cannot forget creates a new way to remember. We change the memory of our past into a hope for our future. – Lewis B. Smedes

Your past is your history but to hold onto the sorrow, pain, disappointment, anger, rage, bitterness, sadness, depression and other negative feelings poison your future. Part of your old mindset may have been to stuff feelings down very deep inside so access would be almost impossible. The way I stuffed the feelings of being sexually molested. But repressed feelings are still there waiting to resurface.

In fact, the more feelings you stuff inside the greater the explosion when they finally erupt. That's the reason some murders are labeled "temporary insanity" because you may truly have no control over your sanity at that moment in time. Not only do repressed feelings stifle your capability to manifest positive things in your life they cause disease and chronic illness. They don't stay in the innermost recesses of your mind. The feelings come out in ways you least expect it.

You can try to force the memories away but, because your subconscious mind remembers literally everything, it is an impossible task. Rather than repress memories and feelings it is best to dissipate them. I view it as letting the air out of an over-inflated balloon. You don't want to pop the balloon so it makes a loud noise and causes a disturbance. You want to just slowly deflate it.

That's what you will do in the exercise of letting go of your past memories and emotions. Not just letting them go but letting them go in love. Love for yourself. Love for the other person if possible. Understanding at a deep level that the emotions are harmful only to YOU -- so you are ready to release them and move forward. You realize that your conscious mind can't let them go but you can consciously direct your subconscious mind to do so.

When you let go of old, toxic emotions and their connections to your physical and emotional body you are healing yourself on all levels. Mental, emotional, physical and energetic bodies are healed when you allow yourself to let go and move forward. Don't allow yourself to be stuck in the past. *You can be what you choose to be.* You can choose to be free of the old negative programming and open to a new way of feeling. A way that let's your soul soar and your body heal.

"I am what I choose to be!"

We've all heard the old adage "resentment is the poison that kills you". It's true. Slowly, surely and purposely it will eat away at your body and your mind. Now is the time to choose a different path. A path that will lead you to new adventures, new choices, new mates, new outcomes and a NEW YOU! "I am what I choose to be" is your new mantra. It's a powerful statement. Say it frequently during the day. "I am what I choose to be!"

Carrying grudges and holding onto old anger isn't affecting the person who harmed you. I know it's hard to let go of it because there is a part of you that feels entitled to feel the way you do. And you are! But the person that you are angry or upset with isn't feeling what you're feeling. They could care less about the emotions you're harboring inside because they are probably unaware of them. And if they are aware, and have done to rectify the issue, they could really care less. You will not move forward in life if you hold onto the old mindset. It is impossible. Why? You won't resonate with positive things and your old programming will hold you back from living the life you were intended to live.

The person or persons who harmed you are not forgiven for their sake. They are forgiven for yours. As you change your mindset it will be less and less important to your ego, the singular "I" that only cares only about itself, that you seek justice. Karma never forgets an address. It doesn't matter if you're the one who brings the karma or not. It is a LAW and it will happen to whomever harms you. And, to you if you harm another. It can't fail. Whether you witness the karma or not is a different issue. But it's there.

I have known a woman for many years and she wished her husband would die for the past decade. She wanted to inherit his millions. She thought she would literally be a *merry widow*. She wasted all of her life, over 25 years, with a man she didn't love or respect because of her love of his *money*. She frequently spoke about wishing he would die, and she felt he deserved it because he hadn't been the best husband in the world. I agree that he wasn't a good husband but she wasn't a good wife, either.

He divorced her right before he died. Did not leave her a penny of his fortune. Instead he left it to his home remodeler and his wife. All of it. To the tune of $10-$15 million. She was furious and asked me if I thought he would receive his karma if there was life after death. My reply was; "Do you think you received yours?" We all get our karma and you don't have to wish it upon someone for it to happen. It may be in a different way, and not exactly the way you were harmed, but it will happen.

For some reason Brad and Angelina came to mind when I wrote the last paragraph. "The way you get them is the way you lose them" is an old adage. I don't know what happened in their marriage but she cavorted with him during his marriage to Jennifer Anniston and then they lived together after his divorce. Six kids later, and a hefty divorce settlement, they are now divorced. I don't know if you noticed how stressed out he looked and how miserable they both appeared to be during their two-year divorce battle, but I did. There was no *happy ever after* for them and the way she lost him, and they broke up, was just as traumatic to them both as it was for Jennifer I'm sure. Karma.

Let go of your past so you can soar into the future! Clean out that old programming and you will be so much lighter, more free, carefree and exuberant than ever before. "I AM WHAT I CHOOSE TO BE!" In the next section we will address how powerful "I AM" statements are because they are truly lifechanging.

EXERCISE FOR RELEASING NEGATIVE EMOTIONS

1. When you get into bed and are ready for sleep close your eyes and breathe in to the count of 4, hold the breath to the count of 7, breathe out to the count of 8. Do this several times but don't make yourself dizzy. This will immediately begin to relax you.

2. Tell yourself "sleep" a few times. Since you have been doing the exercise for a while you should immediately begin to shift into a relaxed and receptive state. See yourself going down the staircase one step at a time and with each step tell yourself "sleep". With every step you take DOWN say the word "sleep" in your mind. Start with the number 15, visualize or mentally repeat the word "sleep", and count down *very slowly*. 15, 14, 13, 12, 11, 10, ...

3. Take a few minutes to totally relax your body starting at the top of your head. You may not need to spend as much time as in the previous chapter's exercise but make sure you are totally and completely relaxed before continuing.

4. Entering the alpha state you are now ready to let go of past negative feelings. You don't need to let go of everything all at once – *toxic overload*. Just tune into the feelings or person you have negative feelings about (allow them to come up naturally or purposefully think of them) and then see, feel, or sense the feelings. You may visualize the emotions as a cloud, feel them as a heaviness in your chest, a lump in your throat, other uncomfortable bodily sensations OR just have the emotion surface organically. Send a powerful intention and a visualization of golden light INTO the feelings as they begin to evaporate and disappear. This negative feeling NO LONGER has any control over you or your future. You have thrown it out of your subconscious mind, allowed it to disintegrate and disappear through your visualization. Visualize as

clearly as possible this emotion dissolving as you state "I AM AT PEACE" and "I AM FREE OF THIS NEGATIVE MEMORY & EMOTION". As you're doing this allow the feeling and emotion of PEACE to permeate every possible cell in your body. Focus on the heart area, or the solar plexus, and state over and over again "I AM AT PEACE" and "I AM FREE OF THIS NEGATIVE EMOTION". Stay in this visualization as long as you feel you need to as you release and fill this area, where the negative thought or emotion was residing, with a golden light. A golden light of love and healing.

5. Now make a mental command for your mind to keep the feeling of this moment in your memory bank permanently AND forever and state this a few times to implant it firmly into your subconscious.

6. After you have done this make the command "IT IS DONE" or simply "LET THIS COMMAND BE FULFILLED". You may then begin to count UP until you reach the number 15 and you will be ready for sleep.

You can do this exercise for everyone you have ill feelings toward if you choose. Don't lump them all together as in "bad childhood memories". Take your time and release them as slowly as necessary so you can really neutralize the negative memories. Try to get to the heart of the issue if possible. Rather than "I feel unappreciated" attempt to find the source of the feeling. Once you do see it as a dark, heavy cloud that becomes lighter and lighter in color and density as you release the negative emotions. Or maybe a heavy or dark feeling in your body that feels lighter, more at ease and at peace. Your subconscious will guide you to the best way to release the past negativity. Trust it!

Do this for several days until you feel yourself becoming at peace internally. You'll know when you feel able to release old, stagnant and useless emotions. You will feel lighter, freer and more carefree as well as positive!

Occasionally you may feel a *hangover* of the feeling, emotions that cause you to cry or even experience a feeling of anger. If that happens it's okay. Just state "I AM WHAT I CHOOSE TO BE" during the day because no one can control you but YOU. They are no longer in charge of your feelings, repressed or otherwise, you are. You are programming those negative things out of your psyche and they have no control over you now. I AM WHAT I CHOOSE TO BE!

If you have meditation music play it as you fall asleep. If not, just allow yourself to feel the power in the statement and use it as your mantra. I AM WHAT I CHOOSE TO BE. Over & over until you fall asleep. When you awake you should feel more positive, lighter and have a more positive attitude about life in general.

HEALING ABANDONMENT ISSUES

Unless you have been able to successfully exit from relationships in charge of your emotions and unscathed you most likely suffer from abandonment issues. They actually are created earlier in life from needs that are unmet in childhood and continue throughout adulthood. They can cause you to attract the same type of partner, usually distant and in control, without you even realizing it until after a breakup. "He's just like the last one!" is most likely how you will feel after another failed relationship. He resonated with you in a level that you have not identified, yet. A level that triggers attraction in your subconscious mind.

If you were not nurtured during childhood you may seek relationships that are somewhat of a challenge where you may wrestle for control or vie for his love. In this way you can prove that you are *worthy* in some way that you feel is lacking in your character. Even women who are the first to end a relationship do so because they have associated being the first to leave as mitigating the pain of a breakup.

For this reason, the following self-hypnosis/meditation exercise will help you heal the inner child who still feels wounded in some way. You don't have to know how the inner YOU is wounded, experience the pain of the emotions or wallow in the feelings – you will just offer your love and support through visualization.

EXERCISE TO HEAL ABANDONMENT ISSUES

1. When you get into bed and are ready for sleep close your eyes and breathe in to the count of 4, hold the breath to the count of 7, breathe out to the count of 8. Do this several times but don't make yourself dizzy. This will immediately begin to relax you.

2. Tell yourself "sleep" a few times. Since you have been doing the exercise for a while you should immediately begin to shift into a

relaxed and receptive state. See yourself going down the staircase one step at a time and with each step tell yourself "sleep". With every step you take DOWN say the word "sleep" in your mind. Start with the number 15, visualize or mentally repeat the word "sleep", and count down *very slowly*. 15, 14, 13, 12, 11, 10, ...

3. Take a few minutes to totally relax your body starting at the top of your head. You may not need to spend as much time as in the previous chapter's exercise but make sure you are totally and completely relaxed before continuing.

4. Entering the alpha state, you are now ready to really heal and support your inner child and change your mindset to stop attracting men whom you have to chase or those that emotionally abuse you. Visualize the innocent and loving YOU at a young age of approximately 2-5 years old. Or, if you have a specific memory of an incident that left you feeling sad or unloved tune into that moment in time. You may see, sense, feel or imagine that time in your young life. As you

tune into the feelings and innocence of yourself at that age take a moment to really look closely, noticing every detail possible. This sweet, innocent, trusting child is YOU and she still resides deep within your soul. Open your heart and let it fill completely with love and admiration for the little girl within. Knowing all of the pain, suffering and hardship she will endure in her life gives you a unique and special bond with her at this moment. She has been strong, resilient and has never lost that innocence in her heart. She has a character and strength that is to be admired, cherished and loved. Take her in your arms and hold her against your chest as you would any small child that needs and desires your love and acceptance. As you do this you can almost smell the fragrance of her hair and feel the smallness of her body. Allow yourself to really let all of your senses experience this special moment. Open your heart and allow your love for this inner child to flow over and out of your heart to her. You may feel she is being surrounded by the love OR that she is merging with your own adult being. *This is a positive experience for her and for you.* You don't have to verbally say anything because there are no words necessary. You don't need to relive her life or any trauma because you both know it's there. You just want to enjoy the merging of the two of you, revel in the strength it gives you, and surround the two of you with an aura of complete love and acceptance. Visualize and FEEL as clearly as possible this emotion of love and admiration for the inner child as you state "I AM AT PEACE AND I AM STRONG" and "I WILL ATTRACT ONLY THOSE WHO WILL HONOR AND LOVE ME FROM NOW ON". As you're doing this allow the feeling and emotion of peace and love to permeate every possible cell in your body. Focus on the heart area, or the solar plexus, and state over and over again "I AM AT PEACE AND I AM STRONG" and "I WILL ATTRACT ONLY THOSE WHO WILL HONOR AND LOVE ME FROM NOW ON". Stay in this visualization as long as you feel you need to as you fill your entire heart area and every cell in your body with love. Love for yourself and for your inner child who will never abandon you, never hurt you and will always be there with you.

5. Now make a mental command for your mind to keep the feeling of this moment in your memory bank permanently AND forever and state this a few times to implant it firmly into your subconscious.

6. After you have done this make the command "IT IS DONE" or simply "LET THIS COMMAND BE FULFILLED". You may then begin to count UP until you reach the number 15 and you will be ready for sleep.

Once you do the exercise it is time to go to sleep. Take some deep, cleansing breaths and allow yourself to relax completely and fall asleep. If you have any lingering feelings you may simply repeat the earlier mantra of "I AM WHAT I CHOOSE TO BE".

Chapter 10 – The Most Powerful Words on Earth

*"**I AM**" two of the most powerful words. For what you put after them shapes your reality."*

These two words "I AM" are so powerful they have the ability to immediately begin to shift your reality. They cause the conscious, the subconscious and the superconscious minds to merge together in the creation of your future. The conscious mind controls your outer world, your analytical mind and decision making. The subconscious is in control of your dreams, the central nervous system, emotions, habits/programs, imagination, creativity, intuition and long-term memory.

"I AM" starts the process in the subconscious mind to begin creating. That process is carried forward and brought into reality by the superconscious mind by holding the desire, belief and vision. All work in perfect harmony to produce positive results!

The superconscious mind is the mind that connects EVERYTHING in the universe. It is the source of ALL knowledge and the place where inspiration, ideas and intuition reside. In order to have access to the powerful superconscious mind you must be in a receptive alpha or theta state, have concise thoughts and use your emotion as the fuel. You will enter a theta state in a later chapter.

> "You cannot fail when you bring the conscious, subconscious and superconscious minds together for creation!"

For now, you will access the conscious, subconscious and superconscious state using "I AM" affirmations. Remember, the subconscious mind doesn't know truth from fiction and when your conscious mind makes the "I AM" affirmation it *commands* it! So, the statement "I AM healthy" will command the conscious mind to bring about the state of health, your subconscious mind will *believe* the statement, and set about the process of becoming healthy. The superconscious mind is the world of "I AM" and it taps into the energy of ALL of the power of the universe to assist you in *being* healthy.

There are many powerful "I AM" statements that you can use for this exercise. I have created a list of statements that you may choose to use if they resonate with you. You may access them by going to: http://laniestevensauthor.com/i-am-affirmations

You can also create your own list, or you may just choose to go with whatever you are *feeling* at the moment. I suggest, when doing the exercise, that you focus on a few statements at a time and use the same ones for a couple of days. You want to have the affirmations firmly anchored into your subconscious mind and that happens with repetition.

You can address anything you have concerns about whether the issues you want to shift are physical, mental, real or imagined. Simply stating "I AM" will start the process of change.

EXERCISE TO REPROGRAM POSITIVITY

1. When you get into bed and are ready for sleep close your eyes and breathe in to the count of 4, hold the breath to the count of 7, breathe out to the count of 8. Do this

several times but don't make yourself dizzy. This will immediately begin to relax you.

2. Tell yourself "sleep" a few times. Since you have been doing the exercise for a few days you should immediately shift into a relaxed and receptive state. See yourself going down the staircase one step at a time and with each step tell yourself "sleep". Start with the number 15, visualize or mentally repeat the word "sleep", and count down *very slowly*. 15, 14, 13, 12, 11, ...

3. Take a few minutes to totally relax your body starting at the top of your head. You may not need to spend as much time as in the previous chapters exercise but make sure you are totally and completely relaxed before continuing.

4. Entering the alpha state, you are now ready to make powerful affirmations always beginning with the two words: "I AM" You can make commands and statements that you record for listening OR that you create spontaneously. Make positive statements designed to create *change* within you. For instance: I AM in a relationship, I AM

peaceful, I AM financially secure, I AM healthy, I AM love, I AM secure, I AM strong, I AM powerful, I AM ready for positive change – you get the picture. The statements you make immediately begin to work wonders in your body and mind creating the conditions to make the statements true! These statements will assist the healing process and begin to fill up the subconscious with positivity. Especially after the previous exercise where you began to rid yourself of negative and program yourself to a different mindset.

5. Now make a mental command for your mind to keep the feeling of this moment in your memory bank permanently AND forever and state this a few times to implant it firmly into your subconscious.

6. After you have done this make the command "IT IS DONE" or simply "LET THIS COMMAND BE FULFILLED". You may then begin to count UP until you reach the number 15 and you will be ready for sleep.

Continue during the day to make the "I AM" statements to yourself mentally or out loud. You have cleared yourself of so much negativity and past programming these powerful statements will revitalize you from the inside out. You can also continue your mantra of "I AM what I choose to be". I am healthy, I am wealthy, I am grateful, I am appreciative, I am happy, I am loved, I am lucky, I am attracting positive things, I am love.

I use "I AM" affirmations all throughout the day because they illicit the feelings I had during meditation and are very calming and centering. I just mentally state them when driving, resting or in-between clients.

Chapter 11 – Special Connections

"Each time we connect physically with another a merger is happening, a merger that goes beyond just a physical connection. The first layer of connection is energetic, not physical."

We are energetic beings and we are ALL connected through what quantum physics refers to as *entanglement.* Your thoughts, being pure energy, can easily utilize that connection to connect you to others energetically using just the power of your intention. When you focus on a person, because we are all connected in this world of vibrating energy, your thoughts are easily transferable. The more *entangled* you are with the person the easier it is to influence and connect your energy to theirs.

In intimate relationships you have a very special physical *and* emotional connection and that's why oftentimes you will feel someone else's thoughts and energy without consciously trying to connect. There was a study done where two people were wired with EEG monitoring devices and placed in a room to meditate together. At the end of the meditation they were physically separated, and a light strobe was shone in one of the participant's eyes, which caused their brain to react. At the same moment the other person's brain reacted although there was no light shining in their eyes. They were still energetically connected.

This experiment was done with participants who were not intimately connected. You can imagine the power of the connection had they been in a relationship, had a physical attraction or been friends or acquaintances. The connection is real. The only thing that prevents people from using the connection is lack of understanding, motivation or not knowing it exists. I wrote two other books about the subject of entanglement and how to use it for love and for sexual interest. Remote seduction absolutely works and so does using the method for attracting a love interest.

For the purpose of this exercise I won't go into all of the details previously written about in the books to control your man or for remote seduction. This exercise will be to strengthen your connection to anyone you choose. You may send love, healing or just enjoy the connection – it's up to you.

You will have a specific location for the visualization for EACH person you connect with during the exercise. Each location will be specific for the person you are visualizing. The place may be a place you have been together, a place of importance to the person you're connecting with OR to you, a place neither of you have been but you would like to go, or a place that brings positive emotions to you. The important thing to remember is that each time you do the exercise you will go to the same place (for that person) that you went to before and it will remain the same.

Why? Because it programs your conscious and subconscious minds to automatically connect to the person when you visualize the place. For instance: In the exercise you visualize a particular restaurant where you were proposed to or has an important memory for the two of you. Each time you use the visualization you will go back to that place in your mind. You won't visualize the restaurant one time and the next time imagine a public park. The same place FOR THAT PERSON.

If you choose someone else to connect with, for whatever purpose you want to connect, you will choose a different place for that visualization. Again, each time you do a visualization you will go back to that particular spot. You can visualize as many or as few connections as you choose but do them separately. Don't include other visualizations just because you are already in a relaxed state of mind and want to save time.

It is *impossible* not to connect to the person and have them feel it on some level. It may be under their awareness, or they may not react to the visualization right away, but they will feel the connection and think of you. I have had people contact me while I was in the middle of the visualization. It's a powerful way to connect. You can send love, healing, have a conversation or just have telepathic communication. *Remember, everything is energy and thought transference is real.*

When you go to your special place and visualize the person don't do it by seeing the two of you – that is like a memory. See the person as if they were standing right in front of you. When I do a visualization, I am looking directly into their eyes so I see only the upper part of their body. You can use the technique to:

- send love;

- influence another person -- should you choose;

- for healing (yourself and others);

- use it for thought transference (love, a promotion, a new romantic interest, a contract that needs signing, a salary increase, etc.);

- use it to sexually excite another person;

- diffuse anger between the two of you, etc.

This is the perfect way to heal another person and you don't have to be a Reiki Master or be proficient at some other healing modality. All that is needed is your attention and your intention.

HEAL ANOTHER PERSON

1. If you know for certain the person has a specific illness you can focus on that diagnosis and location of the area affected. For instance; they have breast cancer, so you see the person standing in front of you and imagine or sense the darkness where the cancer resides.

2. You may use your hands (psychically or moving your own hands) as radiating a healing light in the area and imagine the tissue healing

as the tumors shrink in size until they disappear.

3. Or, you can visualize the cancer as a heavy, dark area that is void of any light. Then imagine a healing golden or white light completely shining through the darkness and brightening the whole area with the healing energy. Again, image the tumors disappearing.

4. You can also visualize a grey aura around the person and see it as mist that is evaporating and moving away from the person. The lighter it gets the healthier they appear.

5. I always envision the person telling me how healthy and happy they are that the condition is healed, and they are feeling better than ever before!

HEAL YOURSELF

I find the best way to heal myself is one of the following two ways and they are both equally effective. Before you begin give yourself permission to heal and let go of the illness.

1. I visualize a white light coming through the top of my head (crown area) and I direct it down through my body instructing it to take away any discomfort, pain or illness. Do this only when you have gone through the necessary steps for relaxation in the previous chapters.

2. I direct my mind to go through my body and locate the area of pain or discomfort. I then see, feel and imagine the pain dissipating or the illness going away. I send white light to the area. I have read case histories where amazing healings have been accomplished doing this and I myself have success stories that are pretty amazing!

EXERCISE TO CONNECT TO ANOTHER PERSON

The following exercise is to connect to whomever you choose. It is important to note that *when you do this exercise you can and will influence another person.* If you don't want to have influence over someone else, then I suggest you don't practice the technique or go through the exercise of connecting. After you finish the exercise *BE SURE TO DISCONNECT YOUR ENERGY FIELDS!*

1. When you get into bed and are ready for sleep close your eyes and breathe in to the count of 4, hold the breath to the count of 7, breathe out to the count of 8. Do this several times but don't make yourself dizzy. This will immediately begin to relax you.

2. Tell yourself "sleep" a few times. Since you have been doing the exercise for a while you should immediately shift into a relaxed and receptive state. See yourself going **UP** the golden staircase one step at a time and with each step tell yourself "*sleep*". Start with the number zero, visualize or mentally repeat the word "*sleep*", and count *very slowly*. 2, 3, 4, 5, 6, 7, 8, 9, 10, 11......all the way up to the number 25 or 30. You will know when you are feeling relaxed and can stop counting.

3. You should be into an alpha state without going through the relaxation visualization for the body. You are now ready to go to the special place you have designated for the

person you are choosing to connect to. Visualize the person to the best of your ability as you *see* as much detail as possible. Eyes, nose, mouth, clothing – everything you can mentally visualize makes it very real. You can use your mental telepathy instead of conversation OR you can have a conversation as you would in person. Make it ALWAYS, loving, kind and pleasant. You don't want a visualization that is upsetting or disturbing. If you are having issues with the person the visualization should have them happy, receptive, glad to be with you and positive. FEEL the connection as you engage all of your senses!

4. Get all your senses involved in this interaction because the more real it feels for you the more the other person is going to feel. And, they will feel it faster. Some readers (from other books) have had an orgasm while using a remote seduction form of this technique. You may even dream about the person because your energy fields will be connected.

5. This simple technique is so powerful that the other person will begin to be *summoned* immediately when you enter the special place when you practice it regularly. During the day you may allow yourself to *daydream* about the encounter to strengthen the connection. It isn't necessary to do this more than once a day and do it preferably in the evening before sleep. The guided meditation I have on my website will keep you connected for one hour and then disconnect you (even if you are asleep). Why? Because you want to separate your energy fields so they don't unknowingly draw upon your energy.

6. After your visualization is complete disconnect from the person and see them slowly fading away in your mind OR if you are visualizing a room walk out the door and close it. Mentally tell yourself to disconnect after the visualization so you don't pick up their feelings and/or baggage.

7. Now make a mental command for your mind to keep the feeling of this moment in your memory bank permanently AND forever and

state this a few times to implant it firmly into your subconscious.

8. After you have done this make the command "IT IS DONE" or simply "LET THIS COMMAND BE FULFILLED". You may then begin to count back DOWN from the number chosen to the number zero. You will be ready for sleep.

I just noticed the chapter number on this subject is 11. The number of intuition and a master number. This is an excellent technique to use for your own healing and for your intuition. Imagine your third eye opening, it is the area of guidance and mental telepathy, and just through your intention you will begin to be more insightful and telepathic.

If you are currently not in a relationship but want to attract a love that you are energetically matched to the following exercise will assist you. Be sure that you have gone through the series of exercises to rid yourself of past baggage, pain and resentment so you can attract someone who will be ideal for YOU.

EXERCISE TO ATTRACT LOVE

1. When you get into bed and are ready for sleep close your eyes and breathe in to the count of 4, hold the breath to the count of 7, breathe out to the count of 8. Do this several times but don't make yourself dizzy. This will immediately begin to relax you.

2. Tell yourself "sleep" a few times. Since you have been doing the exercise for a while you should immediately shift into a relaxed and receptive state. See yourself going **UP** the golden staircase one step at a time and with each step tell yourself "*sleep*". Start with the number zero, visualize or mentally repeat the word "*sleep*", and count *very slowly*. 2, 3, 4, 5, 6, 7, 8, 9, 10, 11......all the way up to the number 25 or 30. You will know when you are feeling relaxed and can stop counting.

3. You should be into an alpha state without going through the relaxation visualization for the body. You are now ready to go to the special place you have designated for attracting love. It can be a place in the

cosmos, a real place, any place except your home. I would personally use the cosmos so it can broadcast out as a beacon to like-minded individuals. Visualize yourself as you stand there in all your radiant glory and imagine a bright, white light sending out rays of light like a brilliant star. As you are radiating light fill yourself with the feeling of love – for yourself and for others. State strongly and boldly: I AM ready for love, I AM ready for a relationship, I AM positive minded, I AM releasing the past, I AM ready for a future with a partner, I AM free of old negativity, I AM ready for a positive relationship experience, I AM ready to accept new love, I AM powerful at manifesting, I AM making conscious choices, I AM ready for commitment......add any other I AM statements you choose.

4. Now make a mental command for your mind to keep the feeling of this moment in your memory bank permanently AND forever and state this a few times to implant it firmly into your subconscious.

5. After you have done this make the command "IT IS DONE" or simply "LET THIS COMMAND BE FULFILLED". You may then begin to count DOWN until you reach the number zero and you will be ready for sleep.

As you gently fall asleep allow yourself to have the feeling of being in love with someone envelope your body. You may imagine them lying next to you, holding hands as you drift off to sleep, or any other pleasant visualizations you choose. Know in your heart, your mind and your soul that this visualization will come true. Have the patience and trust that the universe is delivering the *right* person to you without you having to worry, obsess or fret over the outcome.

It is better to wait for the person you desire energetically than to spend countless days trying to disengage from the wrong person and a bad relationship. And, while you are hooking up with the wrong person (as you may have done in the past) you miss the opportunity to meet someone more suitable.

Chapter 12 – Manifesting Money

When you are in alignment with money it will literally seem to come from every source without you having to do anything to receive it. However, most people live their lives with the *scarcity* and *lack* mentality and it causes fear around the subject of finances. There is no lack in the world of manifesting because it is a mindset of abundance. Abundance in all things – not just money!

I know someone who counts her money several times a day. Literally getting out her wallet and the change in her purse to count it. She has such a fear of loss of her funds that she constantly makes sure her money is still intact. The fear of loss she places on her subconscious mind is mind blowing. Logically how could anyone sneak into her wallet and steal her money? But logic doesn't rule the subconscious brain and she isn't interested in changing her habits.

I probably don't need to tell you that she lives her life literally counting pennies. She's a nurse, and makes a decent living, but she is always broke! She can't make it from paycheck to paycheck without having to borrow from someone or invite herself to different homes for her meals. She's 50 years old so she isn't a college student needing a handout.

Her mindset of lack reflects in her life, too. She can't seem to hold onto a relationship, she attracts ALL the wrong men, she has issues with alcohol as she drowns her sorrows, she lives in an apartment that should be well below her means – in other words, she is a hot mess. Her negative programming is reflected in every aspect of her life.

Fear of money OR anything else that you *obsess* over during your lifetime will be guaranteed to happen. One of the reasons generosity creates more abundance is because only if you feel you have an abundance of resources for yourself can you be generous. Or so your subconscious mind believes. Generosity creates a void that is filled with more money. When you give more – you get more!

I have a friend who lost every dime of his fortune due to overconfidence, arrogance with a little narcissism thrown in for good measure. It wasn't a small fortune that he lost, either. He lost every dime of $250 million and he did it in only 7-8 years. He is living proof that, regardless of how much money you have, you can live above your means. For most of us that would have lasted several generations at a minimum. The interesting thing is that he had no appreciation for his amazing luck and fortune AND he wasn't generous with the money. Perhaps if he had gratitude the outcome would have been much different.

Whether you want a better paying job, an idea that comes to you during the exercise in chapter 13, money that is inherited or given to you, or any other form of the abundance the Law of Attraction is the perfect way to receive it. Once you have cleared out the negativity you've been programmed to believe you will begin to resonate with all of the things you desire. Including extra cash!

To be in alignment you can't allow yourself to focus on the fact that your bank balance is soon to be negative or that you hate the job that provides you with a paycheck. Just like all manifesting you must be energetically aligned. The following exercise will help you imprint abundance into your subconscious so fears around the subject will begin to shift.

EXERCISE FOR MANIFESTING MONEY

    1. When you get into bed and are ready for sleep close your eyes and breathe in to the

count of 4, hold the breath to the count of 7, breathe out to the count of 8. Do this several times but don't make yourself dizzy. This will immediately begin to relax you.

2. Tell yourself "sleep" a few times. Since you have been doing the exercise for a while you should immediately shift into a relaxed and receptive state. See yourself going **DOWN** the golden staircase one step at a time and with each step tell yourself "*sleep*". Start with the number 10, visualize or mentally repeat the word "*sleep*", and count *very slowly*. 10, 9, 8, 7, 6,.....all the way DOWN to zero.

3. You should be into an alpha state without going through the relaxation visualization for the body. Create a special place in your mind where you can go each time you meditate for manifesting money. It can be outdoors in an open field, in a bank, on a luxury vacation, sitting in a new car -- any place that you would associate with having a lot of money BUT not in your home.

4. Visualize yourself in this meditation being able to buy all the things you desire in life.

Living the life of your dreams with no worries about finances. You can even visualize several places or purchases. You're writing a check for a home, you're on a yacht, you're dining in fancy restaurants, taking yourself and your family on super vacations, giving a giant check to a charity you love or anything else that makes you feel WEALTHY. I even visualize money falling from the sky and raining down on me. If you own a business you may see customers lined up and out the door, the phones ringing, or your computer showing a lot of business activity.

5. Use the I AM affirmations to imprint your subconscious mind how lucky and wealthy you are. And, how much gratitude you have as you really *feel* the appreciation. I AM WEALTHY, I AM HAPPY, I AM APPRECIATIVE, I AM ATTRACTING WEALTH ALL THE TIME, I AM BLESSED, I AM ABLE TO LIVE A WONDERFUL LIFE, I AM GENEROUS, I AM LIVING THE LIFE OF MY DREAMS, I AM FORTUNATE, I AM LUCKY.

6. Really engage all of your senses in this meditation! Enjoy feeling that you literally have money coming from every source without you having to do a thing to receive it. Let it put a smile on your face and a song in your heart. You don't need to worry about where the money is going to come from, you are going to be blessed with a gift of financial freedom – enjoy it!

7. Now make a mental command for your mind to keep the feeling of this moment in your memory bank permanently AND forever and state this a few times to implant it firmly into your subconscious.

8. After you have done this make the command "IT IS DONE" or simply "LET THIS COMMAND BE FULFILLED". You may then begin to count back UP to the number 10. You will be ready for sleep.

When you begin to receive financial blessings take the time to express your gratitude and appreciation for your blessings. Do it sincerely, and from the heart, because the more you express your gratitude the higher your energetic field and the more you will resonate with ALL positive experiences.

Do this exercise before sleep and allow yourself an inner smile as you drift off into sleep knowing your blessings have been initiated. All you need to do is continue to have gratitude because it is already done as far as the universe is concerned.

Chapter 13 – Divine Guidance

"Whatever your conscious mind assumes and believes to be true, your subconscious mind will accept and bring to pass. Believe in good fortune, divine guidance, right action, and all the blessings of life." -
- Joseph Murphy

We are all connected to a divine Consciousness. Some call this superconsciousness "God", a "Force", "Divine" or any other name that attempts to explain the power that connects everything in the universe. It doesn't really matter the name you give this superconscious mind. All I know is that it does exist.

How am I so certain? Well, besides the out-of-body experience I had years ago, where I had the amazing experience that will last a lifetime, I use this force daily through meditation. I also am fortunate enough to know that I am an intuitive, although I rarely mention this fact, and I know the ability comes from knowledge outside my data bank. I use the intuition to guide my readers when they send me emails, to create books to help my "sisters" and to offer love and support to those in need.

Yes, I do charge a nominal fee for my books but I don't do work strictly for the money. I offer my love and give back to the universe through my service to others. Even the meditations on my website are not only offered at the lowest price possible but they are enhanced and supercharged with love and empowerment. How? Through my intention and through the spoken word. A picture of a person carries an energy that is strong enough a psychic can hold it and feel the essence of the person – even if they have been dead for YEARS.

So, the power, energy and the essence of a voice is very strong as is the intention behind the spoken words. If I could not do my work with love in my heart for others, I would not do it at all. This is my gift to mankind, no matter the seemingly smallness of the gesture, and I offer it as thanks for the divine guidance I receive.

The exercise I am about to share is one I used years ago but no longer need. You won't need it either after a period of time because in sleep the answers will most likely appear. You can't work on yourself energetically and not have magical things happen. Powerful things that will cause your mindset to change. You don't have to know where the guidance comes from and you don't need to even say it is *divine guidance*. It doesn't matter and it doesn't block the guidance. You will still receive answers. Trust the answers! Sometimes they may not be what you want to hear but the answers are always correct when they are not coming from your own mind.

I believe I wrote about this in another book but I'll repeat it. Many, many things have happened to me that have been due to divine guidance and this is just one of them. I was driving on a highway when I received a *mental message* (that happens instantly by the way) to move over because the car coming toward me in the opposite direction was going to hit me and kill me. Instant message! I was listening to the radio and not paying attention to anything else.

What happened? I stomped on the brake pedal and attempted to scoot behind the car in the right lane just BEFORE the oncoming car crossed the double line. I would have been killed because we were both going 65-75MPH and he narrowly missed me. Divine guidance. That's all I'm going to say about the subject. Trust it when you receive it and it may save your life one way or another.

The name of this book is <u>The Miracle Mindset</u> but very few people believe in miracles. Or, they may believe in miracles but they believe they happen to others and not to them. It all goes back to the fact that you have been programmed to feel unworthy of experiences such as miracles. Positive, wonderous things couldn't possibly happen to someone you may view as undeserving. Well, I've had miracles happen to me MANY times and I am no more or less worthy than you.

I am here to tell you that YOU, the person reading this book, is worthy of having amazing and wonderous things in your life. There is no *"better than"* in the world of the divine consciousness of the universe because we are all ONE and we are all equal. We have different goals, dreams and talents but they all contribute to the whole. I view this as being a cell in the body of the *ALL THAT IS,* and the health and well-being of that singular cell contributes to the health and well-being of the whole.

My connection is no greater or less than yours. I just use mine continuously so it may be like a muscle that is a little more developed. Getting answers from the universal mind or universal data bank is uniquely special and ordinary at the same time. Special because once you do it you will be in awe of it. Ordinary because everyone can do it if they choose. If that makes sense.

Once you realize that you are energy, everyone else is energy, thoughts are energy, the universe is vibrating energy, and everyone affects everyone – you will understand the power of your connection. Until then practice the exercise because if you do the answers will come to you. I promise.

EXERCISE TO RECEIVE ANSWERS

1. When you get into bed and are ready for sleep close your eyes and breathe in to the count of 4, hold the breath to the count of 7, breathe out to the count of 8. Do this several times but don't make yourself dizzy. This will immediately begin to relax you.

2. Tell yourself "sleep" a few times. Since you have been doing the exercise continuously you should immediately shift into a relaxed and receptive state. See yourself going **UP** a golden staircase. It may be illuminating a golden glow or just go up into the heavens. Either way is fine. Don't worry about what is holding it up. It's safe and secure. Begin to go **UP** the staircase one rung at a time. As you go up, and you may be floating up the stairs, count the stairs starting with the number one. Count until you feel totally

relaxed and sleepy. At that point stop counting and continue to the third step.

3. Ask a question you would like an answer to. It can be about business issues, a personal problem, another person or some direction you need in life. Just ask the question repeatedly and as if you are in a trance. Meaning without emotion, expectation, voice inflection or anxiety. Over and over again for a couple of minutes just ask the question. If you start to fall asleep or get sleepy keep going and continue to ask the question. After a period of time begin to descend the staircase.

4. As you descend the staircase see yourself floating down the staircase very slowly knowing that everything is perfectly in divine order and there is nothing to worry about. Your question will have an answer if you don't put pressure on yourself to seek the answer. In fact, as you float down the staircase you may receive the answer. It may happen just before you drift off to sleep. Or, in the morning you may wake up with the answer. If not, you can do the exercise

again the next night. When you trust that the universe will give you the answer you take all of the anxiety out of getting it.

5. Now make a mental command for your mind to keep the feeling of this moment in your memory bank permanently AND forever and state this a few times to implant it firmly into your subconscious.

6. After you have done this make the command "IT IS DONE" or simply "LET THIS COMMAND BE FULFILLED".

Expect to get the answer but don't place an expiration date on the question. Expectation is good because it shows that you have faith in the process of attracting something. Pressure is not good because it shows you lack the faith. You must detach from the outcome on all of the exercises. Trust the process because it works.

The more emotion, feeling and positive vibes you put out into the universe the faster things manifest because you are in an energetic alignment with what you desire. Fear, scarcity, anxiety, depression and all of the lower vibration feelings will block you. When you say IT IS DONE or LET THIS COMMAND BE FULFILLED feel the words and the power of them. This isn't a mealy mouth request. This is a command that is set into motion.

You didn't say *"if the stars are in alignment, the moon is in the right phase and the wording is sufficient"* will you please let me have what I desire. You stated a command to the universe and to your inner-self that this was DONE. Period. No expiration date unless you change your mind. It is in the process of being delivered to you. This isn't amazon.com where you can cancel the order or send it back to them at someone else's expense. Nope. This is a divine command that will be honored.

I ask for guidance on many, many things. Almost everything actually. It comes to me sometimes when I least expect it. Like the story about the almost deadly car crash. Most guidance for me comes in-between the regular thoughts that, just like in your mind, go on endlessly. Like when I'm driving and there is a space of no thoughts. When I meditate and calm my mind. The moment before I fall asleep or just after I awake but before I am fully aware of my surroundings. During meditation when I least expect answers.

I've had a full-on conversation in my mind during a 20-minute drive, asking questions I wanted answers to and immediately receiving the answers, without a remembrance of the drive itself. Things like that you never, ever forget. I have a very dear friend who has received actual audible words in answer to a question. When you accept and appreciate the connection there is no limit to the miracles you will encounter. Expect it. Enjoy it. Savor it. Appreciate it.

Chapter 14 – Creating Miracles in Your Life

"If you don't believe in miracles perhaps you've forgotten – YOU ARE ONE!"

Do you feel that you read about miracles but don't receive them in your own life? Or, have you forgotten to take stock of the miracles you experience on a regular basis because they've become commonplace? Either way, in order to amplify the miracles in your life maybe it's time to *actively* change your mental attitude.

The exercises in the previous chapters are an excellent way to shift your energetic being because meditation creates miracles. Also, if you have gratitude for the things you already experience in your life you open the door for miracles. Without gratitude you become too self-centered and narcissistic to recognize the gifts you were given and how lucky you are in your life. Gratitude doesn't have to be about the big things like a new car, an elaborate vacation or an upcoming wedding. Gratitude is best served over the small things that you take for granted like:

- Having appreciation for your loved ones;

- Having gratitude that you have a roof over your head, food in your refrigerator and enough money to pay bills;

- Appreciating the fact that you are healthy, alive and have people who love and care for you;

- Loving the fact that you have the freedom to choose your lifestyle without fear of being judged;

- Self-love! Loving yourself and the miracle that you are is very important in the manifesting process;

- Gratitude for having the ability to heal your body, change your life and attract a mate ALL using only the power of your mind!

Besides gratitude you must forgive yourself and others for any injustices you feel were placed on you because more than likely they were out of ignorance and not intentional. Even if they were done with intention it is always in your best interest to offer forgiveness. Not for them. For your own well-being! Forgive others so you aren't chained to them forever.

Holding onto negative feelings creates resentment and resentment causes dis-*ease*. If someone else has harmed you there is no point in adding insult to injury by harming yourself with resentment. Sure, it may make you feel temporarily better because you feel that forgiveness is too good for them. And, most likely it is! However, resentment is more harmful to you than forgiveness for an injustice -- much more.

Holding onto pain and suffering causes a victim mentality and you aren't going to manifest positive things in your life while *feeling* like a victim. You can't attract what you don't resonate with so feeling victimized attracts more "*victimizers*" into your life. That door was closed earlier during the exercises and you don't ever need to revisit being a victim again.

"Life is a series of thousands of tiny miracles. Notice them!"

Just through using the self-hypnosis/meditation guides in the exercises at the very least you are creating what science has recognized as "the placebo effect". What is that? Studies have shown that your body has the ability, using only belief, to heal itself. Pharmaceutical studies have shown that in clinical trials if a person believes a placebo has the ability to heal them they have the same rate of recovery as those receiving medical treatment.

Your mind is powerful so don't underestimate the ability you have to attract what you desire and deserve. Even if you have never been able to use the Law of Attraction effectively before now you have the ability to change it – starting today! When you release the old blockages, you have room to replace the negative past with the positive future. **Believe it into fruition**!

You are an actor on the stage of life and whatever you choose in your life to *be, do* or *have* is in your control and power. **"YOU ARE WHAT YOU CHOOSE TO BE"** and I hope you will choose to be a powerful, loving, giving, strong, empathetic woman who embodies *the miracle mindset*. Help yourself and others reach the full potential that life has to offer because we live in a beautiful, magical world. Enjoy it!

Meet Lanie Stevens

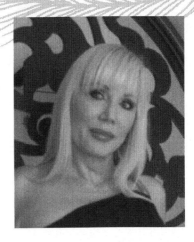

I hope you enjoyed the book and it makes a difference in your life. I have been empowering women for over 20 years using the exact techniques I teach in my books and my "sisters" have been wildly successful.

If you enjoyed the book, please take a moment to write a (hopefully positive) book review on amazon.com. *I appreciate reviews **SO** much!*

Also, go to my website and subscribe for relationship tips, discounts, "freebies" and MORE! http://laniestevensauthor.com

Made in the USA
Middletown, DE
30 November 2019